Affirmation Weaver

A Believe in Yourself Story

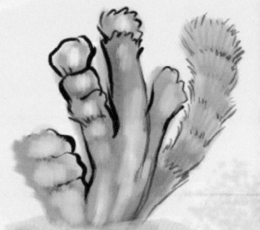

by Lori Lite

illustrated by Max Stasuyk

Congratulations!

You are going to read a story called *Affirmation Weaver.*
An affirmation is a compliment that you give to yourself.
Listen to the wonderful words the sea friends use. Repeat
what you hear to yourself and get ready to feel good!

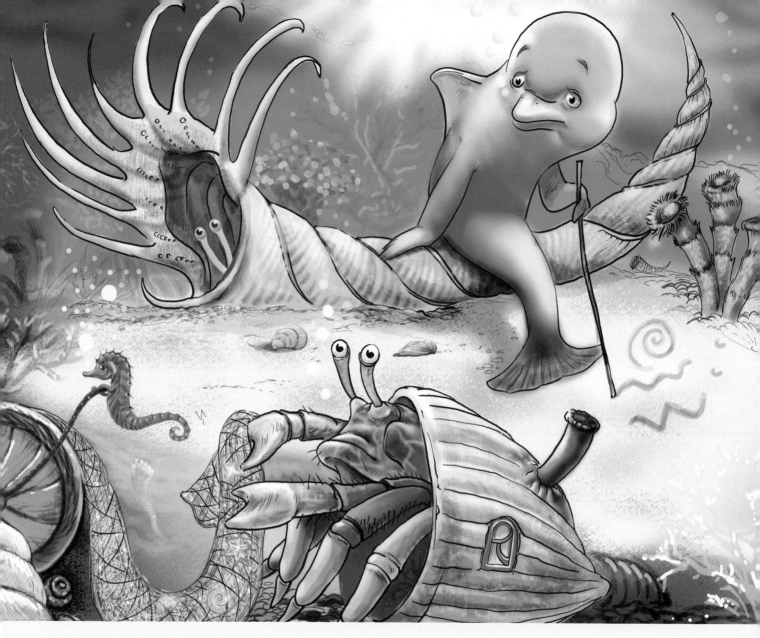

A young dolphin sat at the bottom of the ocean. A hermit crab was weaving a beautiful web made of strands of seaweed.
The hermit crab was known to all the creatures of the ocean as Affirmation Weaver. He was a crab of very few words, but his intricate web brought joy to anyone that took a moment to sit still and enjoy its beauty.

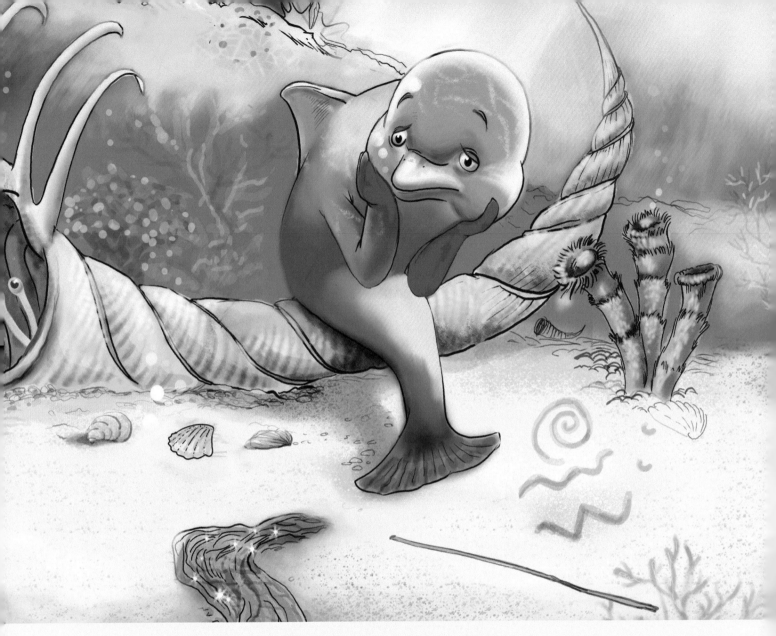

The dolphin was watching the hermit crab weave his web, but he wasn't really paying attention. He was pouting and feeling sorry for himself.
He felt discouraged and sad.

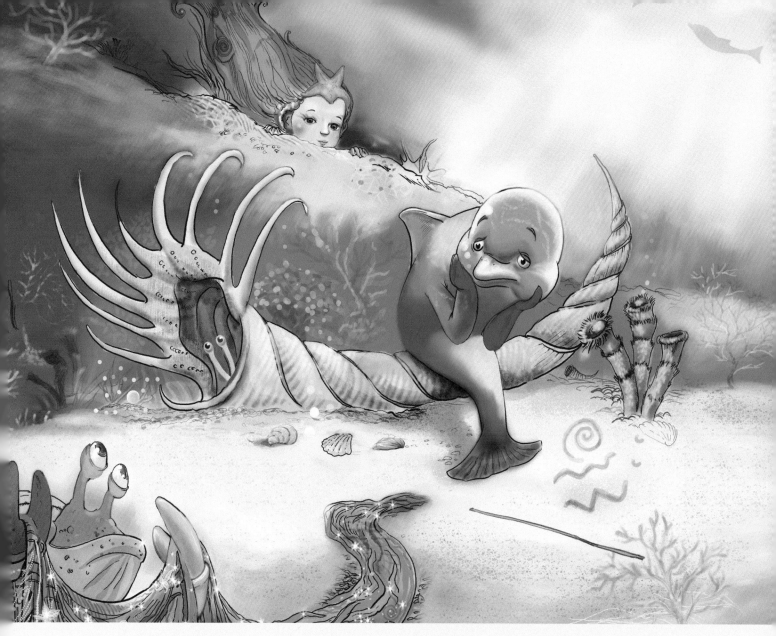

A sea child that had been watching the dolphin decided to ask him a question.
"Why aren't you playing and jumping in the waves
with your dolphin friends?"

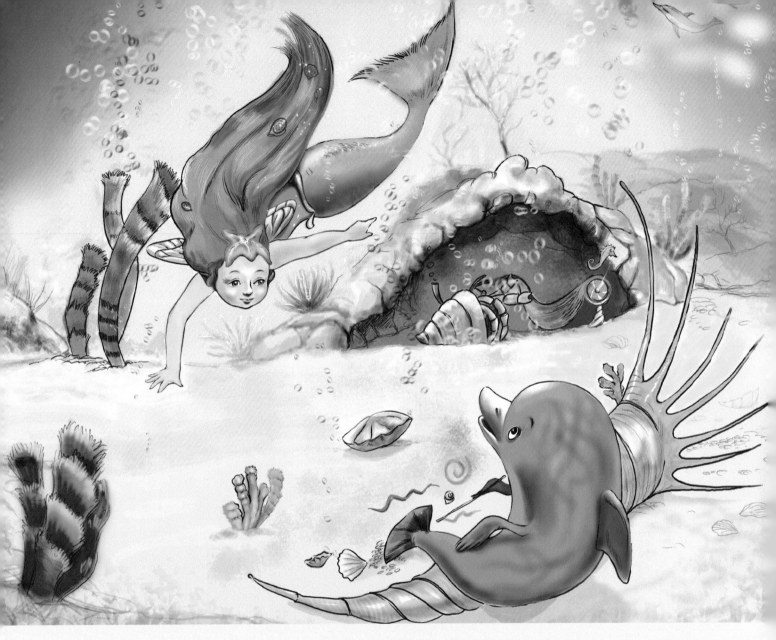

The dolphin told the sea child that he didn't jump as high as the other dolphins.
He didn't think he was smart enough to learn all the fun jumps and tricks that
the other dolphins knew how to do.
The dolphin didn't feel good about himself
and he didn't believe in himself.

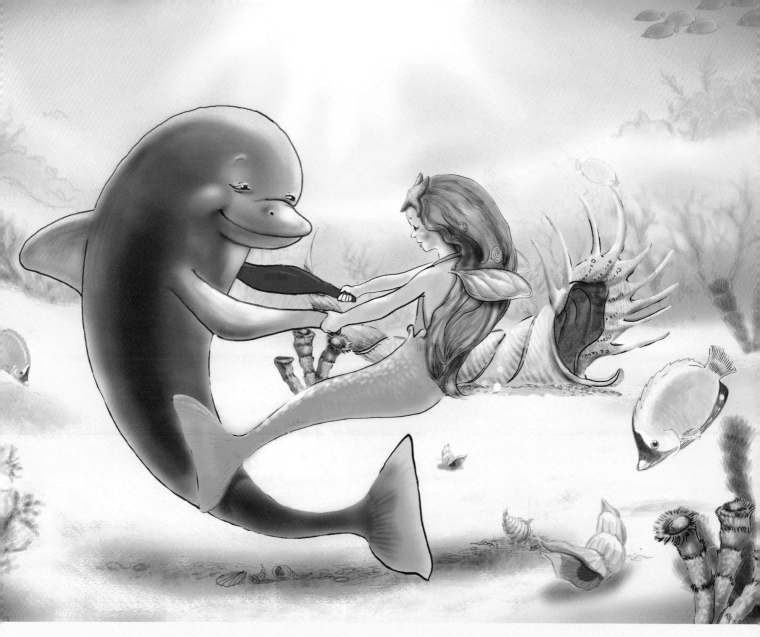

The sea child held the dolphin's fins and looked into his eyes.
"My friends and I feel happy inside. We have a
smile we cannot hide. We say nice things while
we laugh and play. We want to show you
how to feel this way."

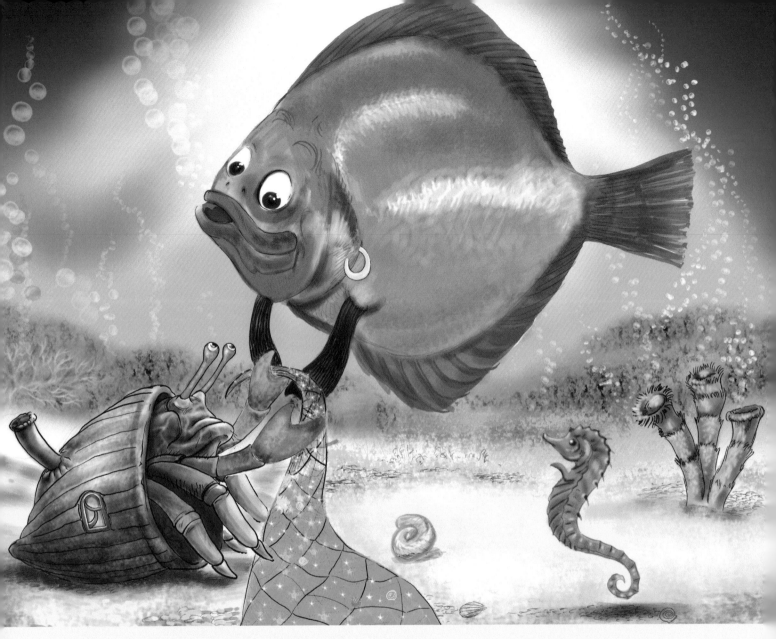

The hermit crab heard the dolphin and knew it was time to weave a different kind of web. A flounder shook the sand off of her head. She placed herself across from the dolphin and said, **"I like myself."**
And with that, the hermit crab scurried over to the flounder leaving behind a shiny strand of seaweed.

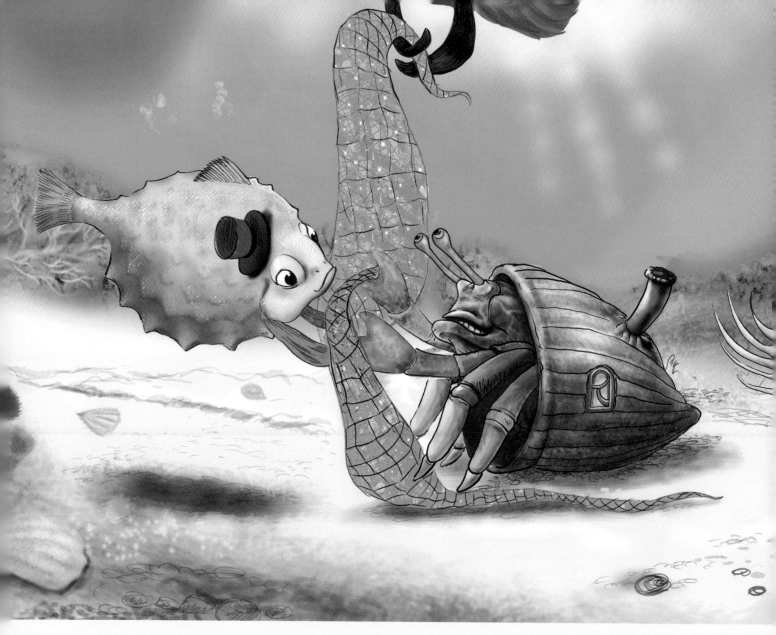

A blowfish hovered into the group. He placed himself across
from the flounder and said,
"I am a gift to the world."
And with that, the hermit crab scurried over
to the blowfish leaving behind a shiny strand of seaweed.

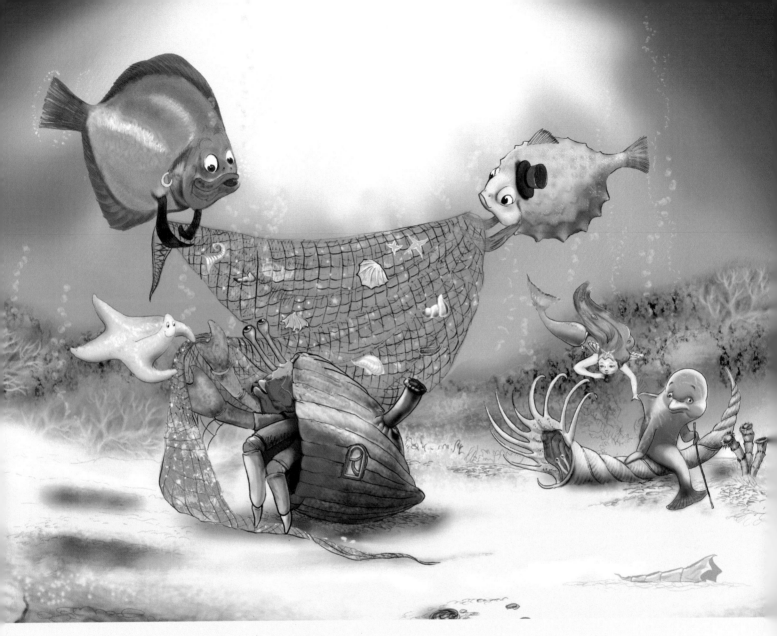

A starfish crawled over to the group. She placed herself across
from the blowfish and said,
"I am creative."
And with that, the hermit crab scurried over
to the starfish leaving behind a shiny strand of seaweed.

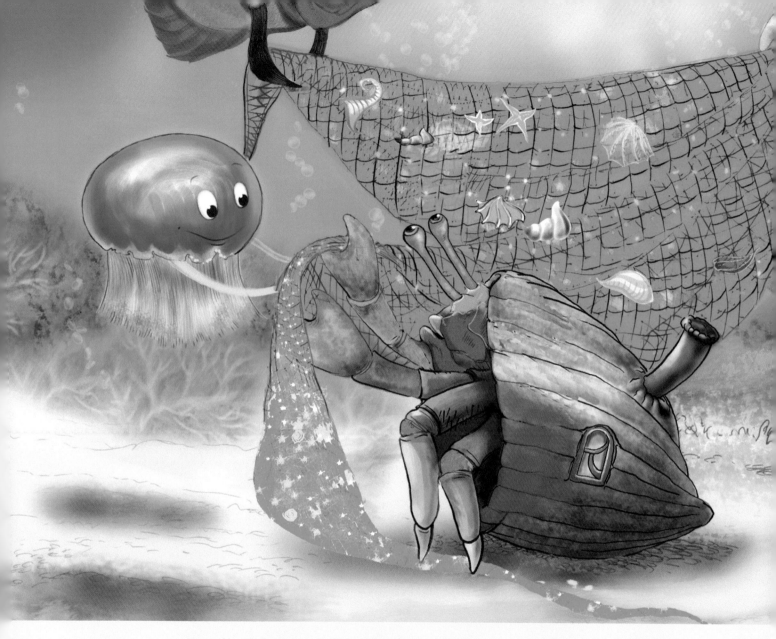

A jellyfish came floating by. He placed himself
across from the blowfish and said,
"I believe in myself."
And with that, the hermit crab scurried over
to the jellyfish leaving behind a shiny strand of seaweed.

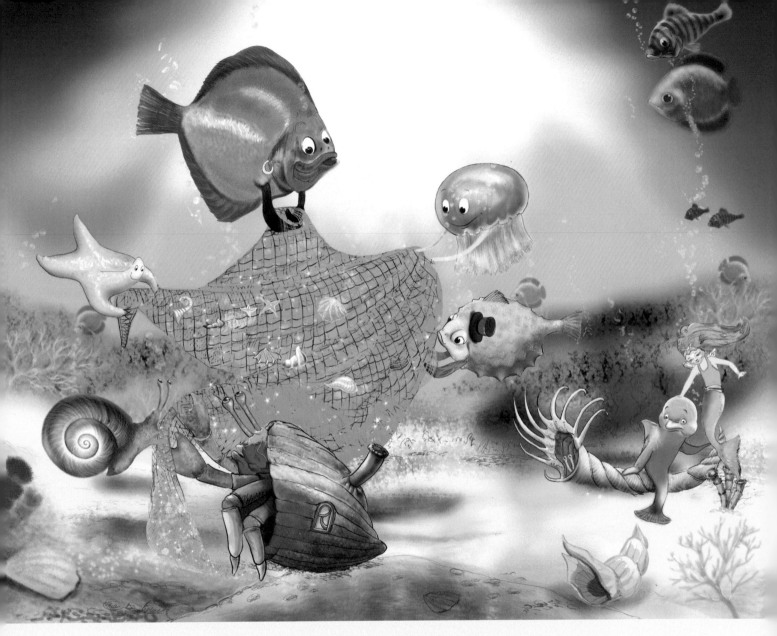

A snail slid slowly into the group. She placed
herself across from the jellyfish and said,
"I learn easily."
And with that, the hermit crab scurried over
to the snail leaving behind a shiny strand of seaweed.

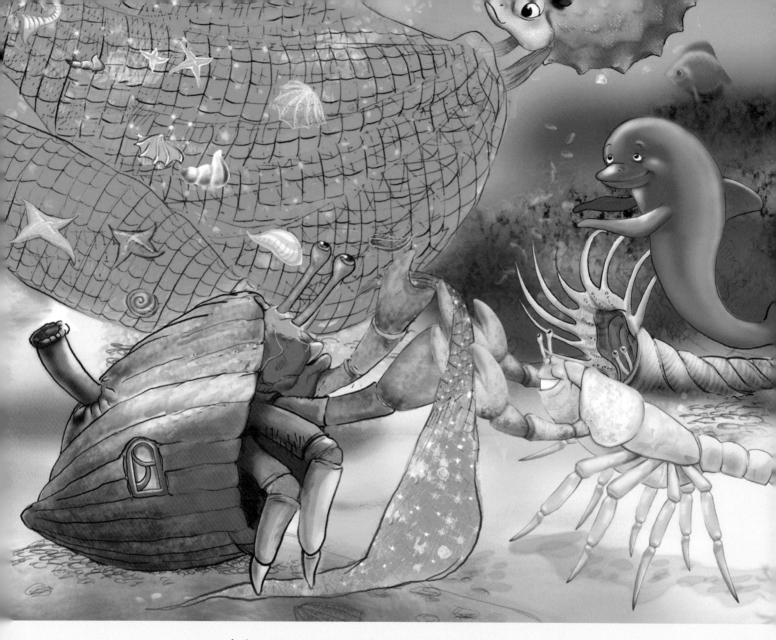

A lobster ventured out of his dark cave.
He placed himself across from the snail and said,
"I am happy."
And with that, the hermit crab scurried over
to the lobster leaving behind a shiny strand of seaweed.

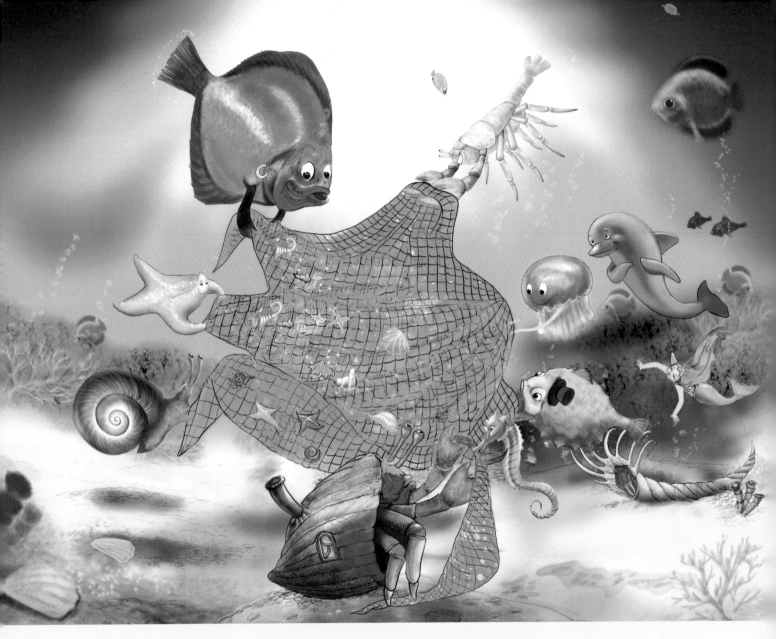

A seahorse entered into the group.
She placed herself across from the lobster and said,
"I am full of life."
And with that, the hermit crab scurried over
to the seahorse leaving behind a shiny strand of seaweed.

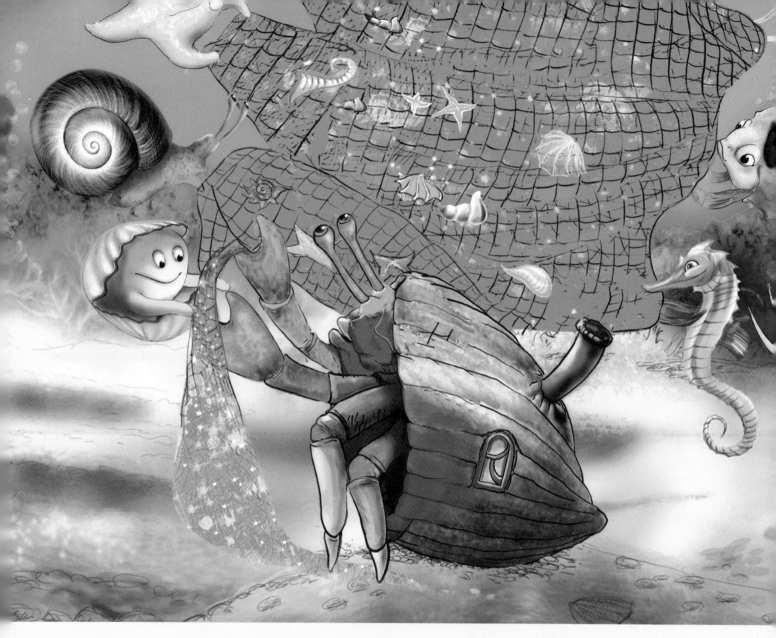

A clam popped up from his underground hole.
He placed himself across from the seahorse and said,
"I can do it."
And with that, the hermit crab scurried over
to the clam leaving behind a shiny strand of seaweed.

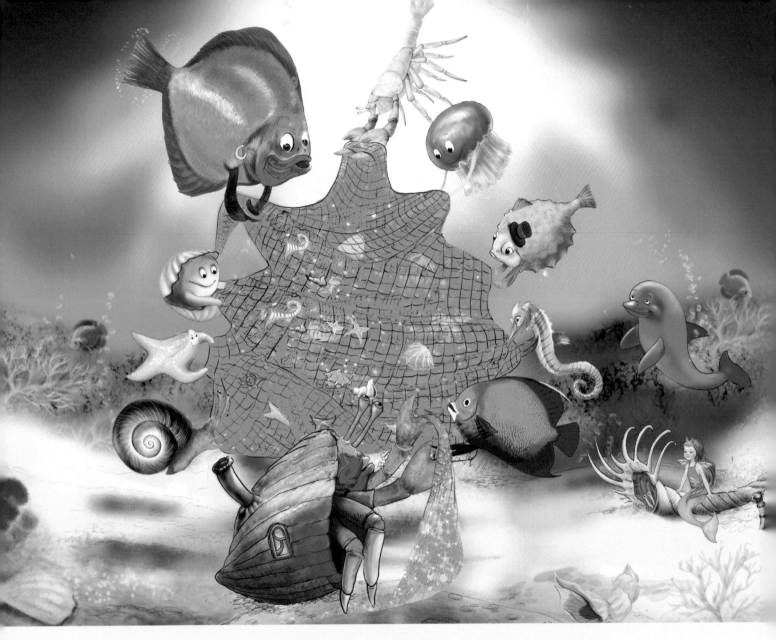

An angel fish glided into the group.
She placed herself across from the clam and said,
"I love myself."
And with that, the hermit crab scurried over
to the angel fish completing the web.

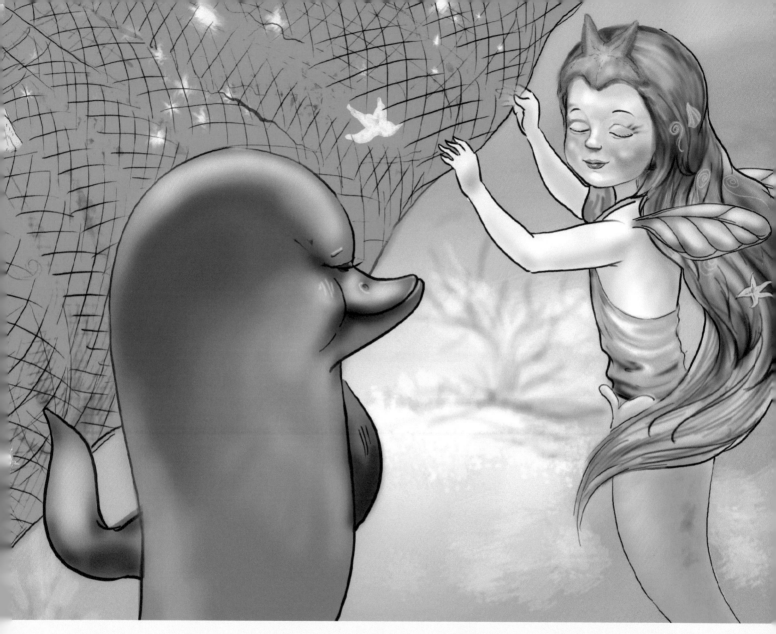

The sea child, dolphin, and sea friends closed their eyes for a moment. They imagined that they could absorb all of the wonderful words they had just shared. They imagined what it would feel like if they could move all of the positive words in their bodies, hearts, and minds.

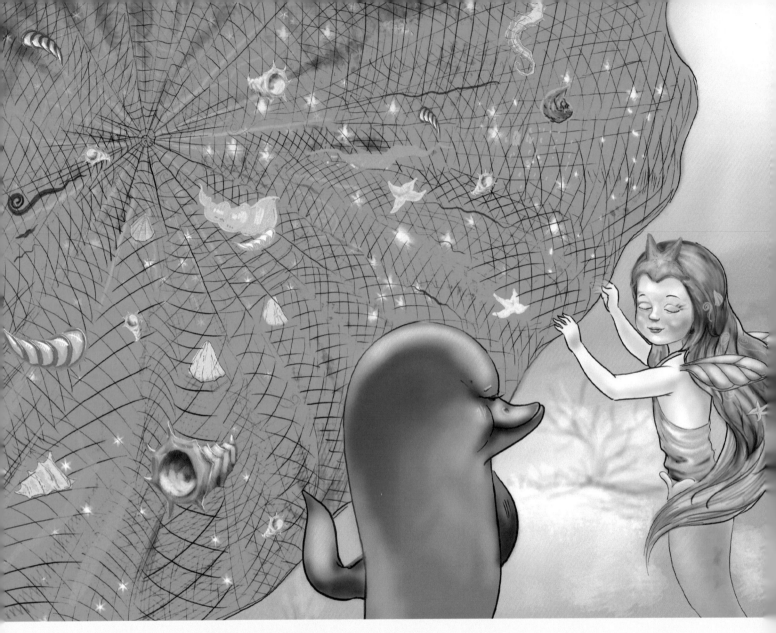

"I am creative. I believe in myself.
I like myself. I am happy. I am full of life.
I am a gift to the world. I learn easily.
I can do it. I love myself."

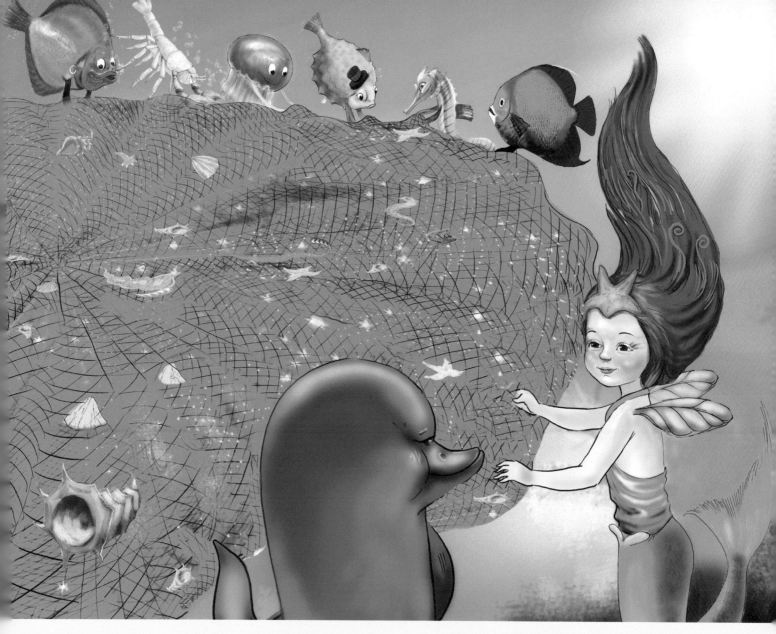

The sea child spoke to the dolphin again.
"Now you're beginning to feel happy inside.
You have a smile you cannot hide.
Say nice things while you laugh and play.
Affirmations help you feel this way."

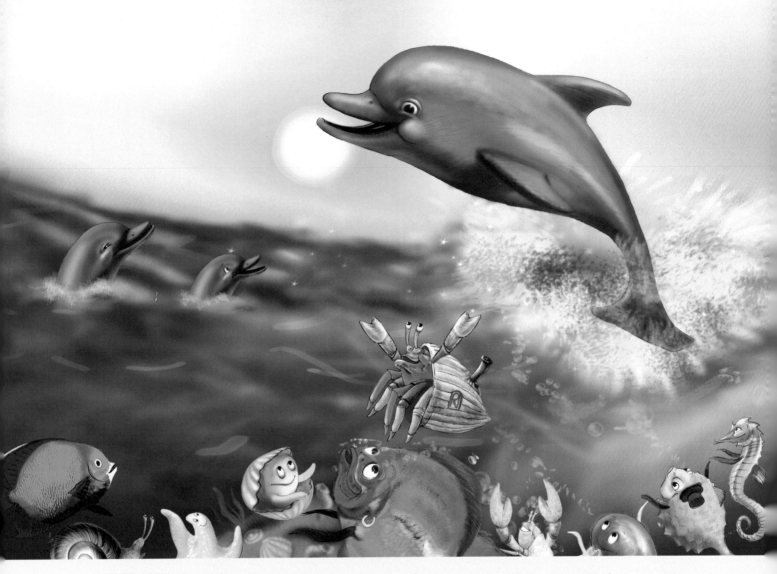

And with that, the dolphin swam straight up to the top of the ocean.
He said, "I can do it", and he jumped high over the very next wave
and landed with a double twist and a splash!
He smiled down at his friends and their wonderful web.

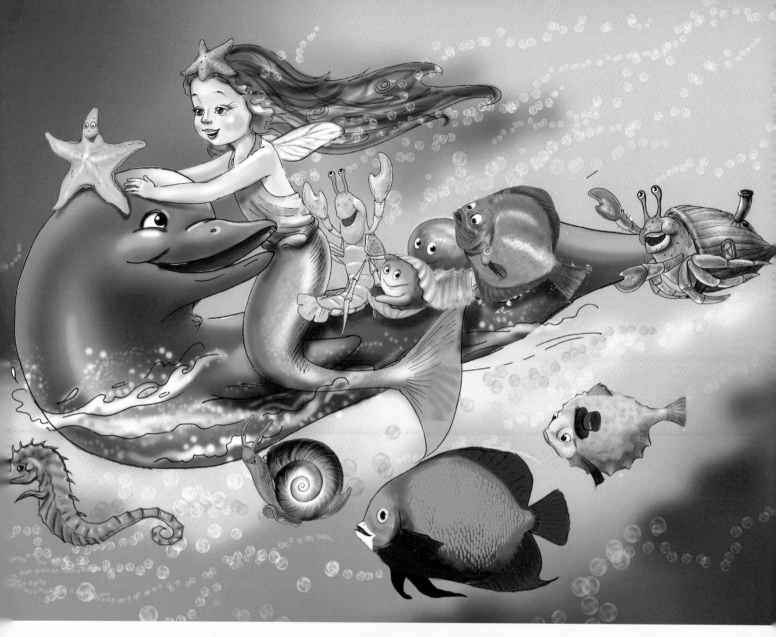

"I love myself just the way I am.
I can do anything I believe I can.
My positive thoughts make me feel good.
Just the way I know I should."

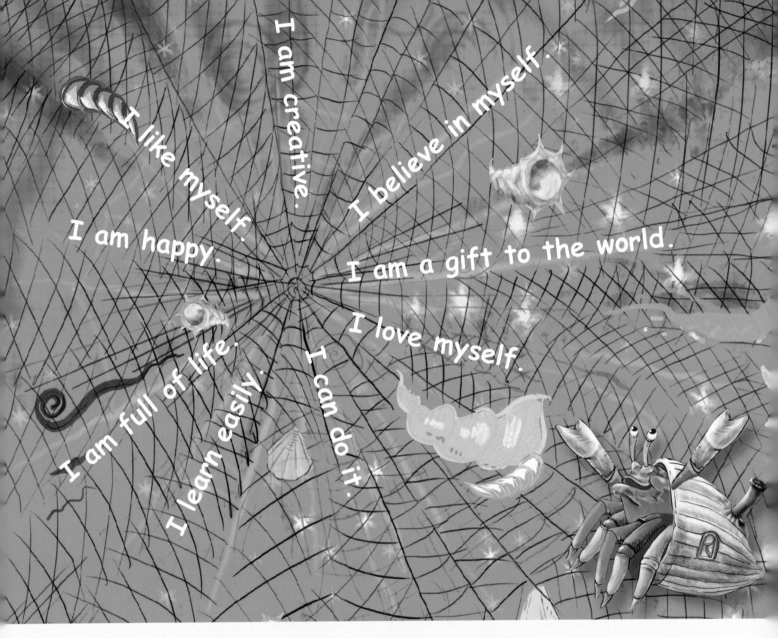

I am creative.

I like myself.

I believe in myself.

I am happy.

I am a gift to the world.

I love myself.

I am full of life.

I learn easily.

I can do it.

And with that, the hermit crab remembered why he was called Affirmation Weaver.

Collect the Indigo Dreams Series and watch your whole family manage anxiety, stress and anger...

CD/Audio Books:

Indigo Dreams

Indigo Ocean Dreams

Indigo Teen Dreams

Indigo Dreams:
Garden of Wellness

Indigo Dreams:
Adult Relaxation

Indigo Dreams:
3 CD Set

Books:

The Goodnight Caterpillar

A Boy and a Turtle

Bubble Riding

Angry Octopus

Sea Otter Cove

Affirmation Weaver

A Boy and a Bear

The Affirmation Web

Music CDs:

Indigo Dreams:
Kids Relaxation Music

Indigo Dreams:
Teen Relaxation Music

Indigo Dreams:
Rainforest Relaxation

Resources:

Individual Lesson Plans

Stress Free Kids Curriculum

**Books, CDs and Lesson Plans are available at
www.StressFreeKids.com**

CPSIA information can be obtained at www.ICGtesting.com
Printed in the USA
LVIW01n0901160917
548564LV00001B/25